Under the Rose-Colored Hat

We are Spiritual Beings having a Human Experience

TRACY CHAMBERLAIN HIGGINBOTHAM

ISBN: 978-1-64184-231-0 (Hardcover)
ISBN: 978-1-64184-232-7 (Paperback)
ISBN: 978-1-64184-233-4 (Ebook)

First Edition

This book is not intended as a substitute for the medical advice of physicians. The reader should regularly consult a physician in matters relating to his/her health and particularly with respect to any symptoms that may require diagnosis or medical attention.

Dedication

To my husband Scott and sons Thomas and Adam for their undying love and support of my entrepreneurial and feminist spirit. I am who I am because I have loved them deeply and they have loved me in return, allowing me to make a positive impact in the world.

To Lynda Rolston Krause, my best friend since the age of four, for funding this book because of her deep faith and our 50-year friendship.

Contents

Introduction 1

Chapter R – Raised Rosy. 3
Chapter O – Overcoming Obstacles 47
Chapter S – Solitude. 53
Chapter E – Empathy and Entrepreneurship . . 57
Chapter H – Healing and Humor 61
Chapter A – Acceptance 71
Chapter T – Togetherness 77

Conclusion 87
Inspiration. 91
Acknowledgements 93
Services Available. 99
About the Author 101

R.

Introduction

Under the Rose-Colored Hat is based on two lessons experienced during an extraordinary time in my life and a challenging time in our nation's history when division, irreconcilable differences and differing perspectives have been sown into society.

This small inspirational story shines a light on the true meaning of beauty, strength and acceptance of oneself throughout life, especially when challenges arise and the need for compassion and acceptance of others in our neighborhoods, states, nation and global environment is paramount. Lessons shared throughout the story will hopefully leave you inspired to change your view of yourself and other people.

Through acceptance and kindness, hopefully together we can make the world a place to witness the goodness of others' actions. If it is true that our perceptions lead to our actions, my hope is that sharing my optimistic experience in the world leads you to see and act the same.

In rose-colored spirit,
Tracy Chamberlain Higginbotham

CHAPTER R

Raised Rosy

Most days of my childhood and teenage years were spent at my Italian grandparent's homestead. A large white farm house with a porch sat at the top of a winding driveway snaking up a small hill to a big flat paved apron for parked cars. A cobblestone barn with thatched roof, next to another smaller barn that use to house livestock in its earlier days, was situated on one side of the driveway. On the other side was a four-stall garage with its infamous basketball hoop and adjoining game room where we played table tennis, if swimming in the large pool behind the Party Barn was getting boring.

The Party Barn was the cobblestone barn converted by my aunt and uncle from an old barn into a rustic, intimate space for social gatherings. The smell of burnt wood hit you in the face when first entering it because half of one wall was a large, old-fashioned fireplace with a wooden beam mantle. On the opposite side of the fireplace was a bar made from old wooden planks with an old-fashioned cash register and small service door where the bartender could deliver drinks to outside guests. We loved being behind the bar pretending to serve grown-up drinks to cousins as if we were already eighteen years old and legal enough to serve and drink alcohol.

Leaving the large party room to go to the aqua pool and multi-tiered deck that overlooked beautiful property, you passed my aunt and uncle's private dressing room, where they stored preferred colorful bathing suits, cover-ups and hip-looking 70s-style avocado green and burnt orange sunglasses. The dressing room had a large mirror and wood pegs drilled into the walls for hanging wet towels. My aunt always emerged from her dressing room looking like Elizabeth Taylor ready for a party. I couldn't wait to be her one day.

Next to the private dressing room were two changing rooms, one for boys and one for girls. My memories stretch back into the mid-70s when there weren't unisex dressing rooms. Since my grandparents had two daughters and one son who produced exactly five granddaughters and five grandsons, equality was important and most likely where my feminist spirit was rooted. They made sure the girls had the same amount of private space as the boys did. There were no favorites in their family, except for my cousin Jeff who seemed to be the one grandchild always allowed to have the biggest serving of macaroni.

The sense of equality flowed out the party barn door over the big sledding hill, past the six tall pine trees that my mother and aunt planted with their father. Continuing past an acre-size tomato field lined with six large weeping willow trees was a slightly smaller garden, producing miscellaneous vegetables and fruits including watermelon, pumpkins, pole beans and potatoes, eventually leading to two forts. My grandfather made one fort for his granddaughters and one for his grandsons. In each wooden fort, which stood triple the size of a typical outhouse, tall and narrow, each had a roof and door. Each sex had typical belongings, the girls had mirrors, dolls, and blankets, and the boys had toy guns, swords and sport equipment. We also knew whose fort was whose from the outside because they were named "Girls" and "Boys," so neither sex entered the other one's special space unless invited.

The changing rooms and forts were the only place on the property which separated the cousins; everywhere else we were equal and together, especially around the dinner table, basketball court, pool, baseball diamond and piano, where any day of the week a different combination of the ten grandchildren played or hung out together. I became an expert basketball foul shooter because I joined in the games my male cousins played together. If they were having a foul-shooting contest or competitive game of H.O.R.S.E., I was up for the challenge. It didn't matter I was a girl; I belonged on that court and had an equal chance of winning against my guy cousins. Today I still possess an accurate foul shot, as witnessed by Syracuse University Coach Jim Boeheim once at a charity event where I sank three baskets in a row to win a prize as he grinned on the sideline.

Since half of my cousins were slightly older than me, the crowd at my grandparent's property frequently included male friends of my male cousins playing a baseball game behind the two barns and in full sight of the pool. Often the girls joined in, because we had the confidence to participate and show off our athletic skills. Many of the friendships in my early days were with my cousin's friends, playing sports in the backyard, driveway or pool. If one of them got cocky enough to attempt and complete a flip off the diving board, thinking one of us girls couldn't do it, we proved them wrong. Fear took a backseat when hanging with my cousins. What they could do, I could do—maybe not better, but I wanted to play. My lifelong love for sports and competitive nature was spurred on by this part of my enjoyable youth.

As summer extended into August, my grandfather displayed his garden trophies on a card table inside their porch next to the kitchen. All sizes of tomatoes, zucchini, pole beans and beets were seen as you passed through the door into the kitchen. If it was canning season, the kitchen windows would be covered in steam from glass bottles cleansed to host the garden's harvest and provide food through winter. In the basement under the kitchen, jars and jars of canned vegetables were stored. Often my grandfather was downstairs checking on his yield and enjoying some dandelion wine. We didn't go downstairs if he was there because we knew he was enjoying himself—or maybe we were too scared to interrupt him. We only went down in the basement to play hide and seek in the winter or to try to spook each other near Halloween.

Everyone knew it was Halloween at my grandparent's house because my playful grandfather always constructed a large pumpkin display with a flying witch to entertain us. Each grandchild could choose their favorite pumpkin to take home and carve. As much as we loved the light in the summer on my grandfather's large lawn, we were equally afraid of it when sunlight hours led to the darker atmosphere of fall. The property was too big to not conjure up scary stories about what was outside lurking around the property. My cousin Tommy would also scare us with stories of ghosts on the property—most likely older Italian relatives who passed away, buried a treasure and were protecting it from being found. We tried to play hide and seek at night, but we just couldn't do it alone, we had to partner up with someone else to keep the jitters away. What's comforting in the light isn't always the same in the dark, and so it was with my grandparent's property and barns.

Dark autumn Friday nights were also a treat as kids when we showed up hungry at my grandparent's house. We had two choices for dinner, the first being homemade pizza with anchovies on them (which we all hated) or deep-fried pizza dough dipped in butter and sugar. Somehow my grandfather always grinned when we choose the fried dough, made into donut-shaped circles, leaving him and my grandmother with their favorite meal. He was sly, but we got exactly what we wanted to fill growing bodies with what we thought was food from heaven. As my grandfather cleaned up the kitchen, doing dishes because my grandmother couldn't walk and stand well, the old-fashioned music from the Lawrence Welk Show played in the background.

In early winter, my grandparent's house was where many ski trips were planned, since my parents owned a ski shop and our entire extended family skied. Visiting Gore Mountain in the Adirondacks of New York State, where my aunt and uncle had a chalet tucked in the woods with a large outside deck, was always a treat. Downstairs, where we kids slept, was pine walls with their very distinct woodsy smell. There were enough beds in one large room for all of us to sleep—again, it didn't matter if we were girls or guys sleeping there, because we were family. Upstairs housed a large open living room and fireplace with quaint kitchen, master bedroom and bathroom. A trip to Gore Mountain and the chalet were some of the special moments of my life. Whether it was tackling a Black Diamond ski trail, going off-trail skiing in the woods with my daring cousins or riding in the gondola, I learned to leave fear behind, embrace the elements, and love the outdoors, most likely contributing to my love of risk.

Returning home from a cold day of skiing, we would settle into a family card game with a fire in the fireplace and Simon and Garfunkel playing on the sound system. Candles burned on the mantel, laughter filled the air and the family was content after a day of exercise and winter escapades. We slept well and got up the next day to do it all over again, until eventually returning home to tell our grandparents about our experiences.

If it was winter and we weren't skiing on the weekends or on special ski trips, you'd find us outdoors on huge snow mounds built by my grandfather, pushing the driveway snow around to clear off parking spots for the family.

Typically, four of us would play on them until lunch was ready. Once we got older, my sister and I would join our cousins walking down the large back hill, through the woods, over a fallen tree to a secret pond that would freeze each winter. There we would shovel off the pond's snow and skate on uneven, bumpy ice, sitting on logs and trees while we rested. When we got cold enough, we trampled through deep snow back to our grandparent's warm home, always heated by wood to a very high degree, where my grandfather wore shorts because the temperature was too hot. We didn't mind since our limbs, cheeks and noses were cold from our outside frivolity. If we were in time, we enjoyed a warm bowl of chicken soup or macaroni. Fresh Italian bread and butter were always on the counter making me a bread-and-butter addict for life. Fresh orange juice was always available to wash it down and keep us healthy.

The love of playing the piano was also handed down through our Italian generations. My aunts and uncles equally possessed musical talent along with a couple of my cousins, so sharing a piano bench was always a family affair. One never knew who was playing the piano entering the house because it could be any family member. Since childhood, I have loved the sound of the piano, even taking a summer of lessons to join our musical family. Just like getting to my grandparent's house, I had to ride my bike to the piano teacher's house for a half-hour lesson and then bike home. I only mastered a few songs which I still play today. I never gained enough experience to play like my relatives.

Besides being a home where food, trips and fun was had, my grandparent's home was also a safe haven in many ways. Never complaining about being a child of divorce at the age of ten, my grandparents and aunt took it upon themselves to open up their home to my sister and I as a safe haven from sadness and stress. If we felt we needed to escape home environments once both our parents remarried, we could jump on our bikes and ride to our grandparent's house where there was always someone to talk to—especially my grandmother. Due to severe arthritis, she sat most of the day in a chair watching television, praying or talking to whoever showed up in her living room. Everyone knew they could find "Minnie" there with pink rosy cheeks, gentle smile and a tender heart and ears to listen. My grandmother was a beloved woman to everyone who knew or met her including my mom's old high school boyfriend, who never stopped visiting her. Childhood friends, college roommates, old boyfriends or girlfriends of my cousins, all visited my grandmother. I imagine she was like visiting a saint where you could discuss anything on your mind without judgment.

She and I had a very special relationship. When she had to move from the living room chair into her bedroom due to declining health, people still visited her bedside. One day she told me to look through her jewelry case to take any of her treasured pieces. She wanted me to have them before anything grave happened to her. A darkened golden locket with a photograph of her and my grandfather just before they got married was my favorite piece. Because Minnie always wore rose-colored clothes, I also took a sparkling rose heart with old-fashioned gems in it to wear and to remember to act like her as often as I could, which meant being kind, friendly, loving and caring. It remains in my jewelry box today and one of my prized possessions.

Years later, after I was married, I attended my husband's grandmother's graveside funeral when the presider said, "If you love someone and they die, the best thing you can do is take the quality you like best about them and inter-twine that quality into your own spirit. By doing this, they live on through you." When my grandmother died, I remembered this advice and intertwined Minnie's happy disposition into my spirit. I have carried her forward in that way in both my personal and entrepreneurial life. Equally special was getting married on my grandparent's 60th wedding anniversary on September 29, 1989 and having her in atten-dance, since my grandfather had died earlier that year.

It wasn't until later in life, when the #MeToo Movement surfaced with stories of sexual abuse and harassment, that I realized that my grand-parent's home had also been a refuge for me and my sister. We lived next door to a married neighbor who exposed himself to us anytime we needed to borrow sugar or flour. My sister and I would fight about who had to go next door and often times we went together to make sure the other one was safe. We never told our mother because it was too embarrassing a subject to bring up or discuss. Whether we appeared at his door, walked up the stairs to the home's deck or was inside his daughter's bedroom, he exposed himself unexpectedly. We were lucky he never touched us. Now I believe leaving our house and spending so much time at my grandparent's house was an escape from this pedophile that we had no control over.

Other difficult situations dotted my upbringing, including the night of November 7, 1973. It was the night of my 9th birthday, so my parents took me, my sister and a boy named Brian Bean, who was staying with us while his parents were out of town, to a restaurant to celebrate. After dinner we came home, lit a fire in the old 1762 colonial fireplace, opened presents in the warmth of the flames, played a game and went to bed. It was a happy day until I was awakened in the middle of the night by my parents rushing my sister and I out of the house because our home was on fire. Luckily, our dog woke up our guest, who ran upstairs and shook my parents awake. They moved quickly across the top of the house to our bedroom to get us. We all ran down a second set of stairs and out the back door to safety.

Alarmed neighbors turned on lights and welcomed us into their homes. We slept overnight at a neighbor's house while our parents spoke to police and tried to figure out what happened to a house that they had spent five years of time and money repairing and renovating. The weeks that followed found the four of us staying in houses my aunt and uncle owned around the lake while our house was fixed. It took an entire winter and into the summer to return home. I'll never forget the first night sleeping back in my old bed and bedroom. It was a hot July night and all I could smell was charcoal and smoke residue still trapped in the house's beams. I have hated the smell of smoke ever since because it reminds me of this traumatic incident.

To say my life began on a colorful note is an understatement. Not only was I lucky enough to be brought up in a warm and caring extended family, on my mother's Italian side, but also by my father's parents, sister and cousins. My paternal side of the family was the Chamberlains who were equally as warm, generous, humorous and kind as the Italian side. My insatiable need to hug everyone, exclaim my love for my sons every time we talk, and

laugh easily at stressful and joyful times came
from them.

My paternal grandfather named "Bopey"
was a joyful man and oldest of seven boys.
His house sat on "Chamberlain Hill," a large
steep parcel of land, bought by his father with
acre plots given to each son. My grandparent's
ranch-styled, pale yellow and white house, with
birch trees dotting the front yard and a huge
garden lining the back, was built by my grandfather to house him and my grandmother after
work in the glove factory and retirement years.
Often the entire Chamberlain gang met behind
my grandparent's house for large family clam-
bakes and endless Pitch card games. They were
a happy bunch of people who overwhelmingly
produced smiles on my face whenever I was in
their company.

Bopey and Grammy Chamberlain's house
was an hour from my home but easily accessible

on holidays and week-long summer vacations where my sister and I stayed with them watching soap operas on television, on hot summer days, after swimming for hours in our great uncle's pool across the street. We were spoiled with large amounts of chocolate mayonnaise cake and other sweets that made visiting these grandparent's house seem like Christmas every day. My sister and I adored them and our extended Chamberlain relatives. God knew what he was doing when he balanced my early life out with two differently-cultured but equally loving and kind families.

I believe each person is born into a family to witness, learn and lead by examples we experience, see and feel, whether they are positive or negative lessons. No one's life is without fortunate and unfortunate instances. Experiences mold us into the person we become for good or bad. Although from the public's perspective, my upbringing was wonderful, filled with the good fortune of growing up on a beautiful lake, being a daughter of popular physical education teachers, coaches and ski shop owners, vacationing in cool places, having food on the table and living in a historic house, they couldn't see that I also survived living next to a pedophile, was traumatized by a fire, experienced two robberies after moving back in to our home after the fire, and eventually living through multiple parental divorces. But the way I look at it, my life has been a blessing and balanced pretty evenly, because the good times outweighed the bad experiences and made me a strong, independent, faith-filled woman who looks through rose-colored glasses and sees life as a glass half-full, not half-empty, experience.

Influential Women

In the midst of my upbringing, I was especially blessed to witness three generations of women whose example in love, faith, and beauty impacted my feminine self in even deeper ways. Whether it was choosing my favorite cream pie for Minnie to make for my birthday, joyfully laughing with my other grandmother, Ginny, attending Catholic church services with my mother or listening to Christian music with my aunt, watching a majority of the women in my family work in their own businesses or being mentored by successful business women, I grew into a woman who appreciates other women.

The wonderful thing about my parent's divorce was eventually having two other adults to add to my parents list. Thanks to my Dad, his marriage to my stepmother, JB, meant becoming a leader of a blended family comprised of eight siblings, six girls and two boys, which naturally placed me in a position to become an empathic giver, concerned about the welfare of others.

Also, being shaped by female family members who spent time ensuring they looked and dressed well, as generously as they gave to those in need within the community, set me on a solid path to model them. Born with a perfectionist personality and good sense of my self-image once out of college, I dressed in beautiful clothes with painted nails accompanied by makeup with a fashionable haircut to guarantee my appearance matched the work environment, leader's expectations and corporate setting. Healthy eating and exercise were essential parts of my routine, just like the women in my family who lived into their middle and late eighties.

After becoming a woman entrepreneur, a quarter century ago, I even took my appearance one step further, dressing in my company's brand colors of black, fuchsia and light pink. A brand color is the color or colors a business chooses for their logo and corporate image. It is used repetitively to have consumers remember them. If you were asked what color McDonald's arches or the color of Starbucks coffee cups are, you probably know the answer, which according to business principals makes you more likely to remember the company and buy from them.

I once heard if a woman is smart promoting her business, she should be dressed to be remembered, so wearing my corporate brand colors made sense. When I created my second company dedicated to helping women, I picked brand colors to represent three women—my maternal grandmother, paternal grandmother and myself. Always wearing black to look classy and formal when conducting business, I made black the essential color of my background images. Black was brightened up with fuchsia because Minnie wore rose-colored pink dresses and Ginny wore red. It was imperative that my logo colors reflect the seriousness of my mission to help women in business and reflect my wonderful grandmothers who were instrumental givers of love.

To understand the depth of this story and the experiences leading me to the lessons I witnessed the past few years, which are the core of this story, you need deeper insight into the females that enhanced my world and carved me into a woman who experienced these recent lessons.

Patricia

Life began three weeks later than it should have to an artsy mother who also had a passion for teaching and playing sports. Standing a whopping 5'1" with an energetic love for competitive sports, blended with an intellectual appetite for the arts, my mother passionately chose a career path that moved her. Right out of the college gate, she taught physical education and coached some boys' sports. If DNA transfers eye color, skin tone and height from parents to their children, then the feminist career gene in my system surely stems from her belief that she could coach boys in the late 1960s.

When I was growing up and after her physical education teaching years, my mother primarily taught dance to hearing impaired students at the New York State School for the Deaf. Like most people, I didn't understand how deaf students could hear the music in order to dance, but later learned they could feel the beat through the floor. Because Patty always loved dance, it made sense for her to leave the competitive sports environment and become a dance teacher for this special community of children and teens. I am not sure if people are born to love the things they do, like the arts, sports or business, or if it is something people are destined to do because that's what God chooses. Even though my mother put me and my sister in ballet and tap dance lessons during our childhood, because that is what she liked, our dance careers came to an end when we became teenagers more interested in skiing, swimming and running. I suppose we were missing her artsy gene.

Although none of Patty's dance students ever went to the New York City Ballet, they did land on many stages across the state and country in Special Arts Festivals. Once in a while my sister and I would enjoy a performance of theirs and also a production of the Syracuse Symphony when they came to our hometown. It was important for us to listen to cultured music no matter how boring it seemed to us at the time. We were treated to this live chamber music because my mother was also a volunteer, providing coffee and cookies for the musicians.

Inviting and cooking for diverse groups of people at our house was a regular occurrence. My mother relished cooking and serving five-course meals, giving her and her guests enough time to truly enjoy and share the evening together. My sister and I often joined in the merriment. Around the table would be a mix of deaf students, gay artists, Catholic priests, blue collar factory workers, African American student teachers, neighbors, musicians, dancers, and coaches. I learned at an early age that everyone belonged at the table and the atmosphere was more enjoyable when it was multi-cultural. My mother was liberal and open-minded and demonstrated kindness to others through food.

Whether teaching my sister and I to ski, swim, waterski or sail a boat by the time we were ten, taking us on summer trips to Cape Cod on a limited budget, or ensuring we became financially independent women, my mom gave us some of the best lessons and memories in life.

Elaine

My mom's sister Elaine was not only my aunt, but my namesake and godmother. I discovered we had similar genetics in terms of interests in business and entrepreneurship. Elaine was a more traditional daughter to my Italian grandparents, choosing to stay close to home instead of going to college and marrying her high-school boyfriend, who became a physician like his father. She invested her husband's paychecks into real estate or restaurant holdings, making more money for their family. On any warm, sunny summer day, she came out of her half of the big white farm house, she shared with my grandparents, dressed to the nines with her jet-black hair curled and laying on the collar to a suit accompanied by a silk top, gold cross, and high heels as she waved goodbye to me and my cousins because she was setting off to conduct business. Her sleek Mercedes sparkled in the sunlight as she drove away. A couple hours later, she returned from her appointments, joining us poolside for a chat and coffee. She was so energized running businesses. Every time she drove out of the driveway, she cemented my interest in following in her heels.

Although Elaine rubbed elbows with the socially elite in town through real estate, restaurants and her husband's practice, she was known for her generosity and compassion, giving jobs to people who needed an opportunity and money to work and live. Whether the employment opportunities were in the food service industry, construction or manual labor around her properties, she offered them to her nieces and nephews, friends of her children and people who needed money.

She even invited strangers to join her family for dinner. I'll never forget one Thanksgiving sitting across from "Herbie" the typically homeless man who hung around my aunt's downtown property. He had no teeth, scrubby facial hair and wore ripped clothes. He sat right in the middle of my aunts, uncles, cousins, grandparents and siblings. He was one of us that year. The memory of him across the table—having a hard time eating his food properly because of a lack of teeth—always stuck with me, along with the generosity of my aunt for inviting him.

If people judged my aunt only by her clothes, cars, and business dealings, they missed the best part of her; her kindness, compassion and big-heartedness.

Dona

My dad's sister Dona was my other aunt who studied nursing at Vassar Hospital. She never graduated because she met a sailor who swept her off her feet. After getting married, she had a job working in Johnstown Hospital helping where she could because she loved taking care of people. As her life continued, she worked in my parents' ski shop, other entrepreneur's stores and even taught blind people to ski. She was never monetarily wealthy like my other aunt, but that never mattered to her or to me. She worked hard at every job she held and contributed to the household income.

She has the prettiest blue eyes and deepest dimples, always accompanied by a joyful laugh. I knew she loved me, almost more than anyone else, by the way she treated me all my life. She always dressed in well-coordinated clothes, dyed and permed her hair and never left the house without makeup until she was 80. Her ears were pierced, and she wore necklaces, often a cross, and multiple rings on her fingers. Her crystal blue eyes sparkled and there was something about her that makes my heart sing. She is a woman full of deep faith and most importantly, joy and love for her family, and spent any spare time writing religious poems for a series of religious and inspirational books. A bookshelf in my house carries a collection of books filled with her special writings. Perhaps my love for inspirational writing was encouraged by my Aunt Dona's love for God as seen in her poems.

Dealing with partial blindness later in life, Dona also taught me—through many deep conversations in her quaint apartment after her husband passed away—that she had it better than most people. Losing eyesight in one eye and having to withstand monthly shots in her seeing eye allowed her to envision loving her life, because she knew life could be worse. Never one to complain, her zeal for believing life was good gave me the strength and perspective needed when times were tough in my life. I've never met a person so grateful for her simple, blessed existence than my Aunt Dona. Through the lenses of her eyes, I saw mine the same way, especially when hardship occurred.

J.B.

The other woman who inspired me to look good and dress well no matter what the budget was my stepmother, J.B. After my parent's divorce, my father met J.B., who had three daughters. Together they created a Brady Bunch of their own by blending three blonde stepsisters Chris, Mar and Beth, with my dark-haired sister Jill and I. Eventually they gave us a sister Bre and two brothers Chad and Jake. Together there were eight of us spanning nineteen years. I was the proud leader of this happy, mixed family posse. The only way to tell we weren't related 100% was by our hair and eye colors—other than that we were family. In terms of birth order, there were six girls before the two boys came along, giving me the lead role of the group and making me an expert of leading girls, which played out in my career.

Our mixed family worked because J.B. was a fun-loving, kind and humorous woman, which helped blend our combined family. Ahead of her time, she lived holistically and was a yoga instructor when my father married her and before the world appreciated health, homegrown food, and holistic practices and perspectives. Her black hair turned snow white when she was in her 40s, giving her a stunning look, which perfectly complemented her pale Canadian skin and soft hazel eyes. J.B. never came downstairs in the morning without makeup and combed hair. She wore colorful loose clothing which matched her comforting disposition.

She was beautiful right up until the day she passed away from Alzheimer's disease, making sure to have on rouge, foundation and combed hair. My stepsisters made sure J.B. looked as beautiful as she always had so her looks didn't die along with her memories of us. Even the hospice nurses complimented her beauty as they took care of her. She remained grateful for everyone's care throughout the entire disease, which doesn't always happen to patients with this illness, proving her beauty also laid deep inside her spirit.

Lynda and Geselle

Balancing out the female relatives who graced and shaped my life were two best friends over a lifetime, with one of them even providing the seed money for this book. Although I don't remember meeting Lynda at the age of four in nursery school, she and I were destined to be lifelong soul sisters before we were born. How else do you explain a fifty-year friendship that spans childhood sleepovers, coming-of-age memories and even early career moments in the big city of Philadelphia, to empty nest moments shared across the country after our children left our homes? You can't. My heart hopes everyone reading this book has that type of long-term sister-friend in life.

It wasn't until junior high school science class that my heart connected with an Italian girl named Geselle who walked into class and sat near me. We hadn't met in elementary school because we came from different parts of our city, but with only two junior high schools, students met others in seventh grade. Once together, Geselle and I discovered we were distant relatives and our mothers were friends in high school—another indication that DNA can flow between mothers and daughters. Geselle and I didn't know we were related until we became inseparable along with Lynda by our sides. Sometimes your dearest soul sisters teach you as much about life, looks, career and yourself as your relatives do.

Olive and Peg

If it wasn't enough that my female relatives and friends presented themselves in their best light, my perception of what I should look and dress like was then influenced by stylish smart women in my early professional career.

Olive was in her late 70s when I met her, standing at a high school event with her beautiful long, white hair up in a bun. Introduced to me by my Aunt Elaine, Olive was the first female President of the Oswego Alumni Association at State University of New York at Oswego, her alma mater. Olive was also a longtime friend of my family who took a liking to me immediately and wanted to mold my sixteen-year-old self into a young female leader. Somehow, I was gifted with this "fairy godmother" who not only lifted me up and gave me essential leadership experience, but also helped me secure my second job out of college working in the same organization she was affiliated with as a trailblazer.

Everyone in my hometown knew Olive. She was an amazing woman married to one of the owners of a large, successful company and an active member of our school Board of Education and a prominent volunteer in the community. She owned a beautiful white colonial house on a busy corner near our high school. She worked on her hands and knees in her beautiful garden as hard as she worked leading companies and boards. In fact, years later she would die peacefully tending to that garden, probably making her happiest of all. Any time I saw Olive she was well dressed in a business skirt and suit jacket with glasses, lipstick and a smile. She never stopped working or looking good until the day she died. She mentored me, and in doing so impressed upon me her own personal dress code and style.

When I landed the job Olive helped me get at SUNY Oswego, it was working for a strawberry blonde, forty-year-old Executive Director named Peg, who dressed beautifully. I only remember Peg dressing down once, when she took the staff out waterskiing one summer afternoon to thank us for working an entire special event weekend. Peg was a fun-loving, detailed-focused boss who taught me to be the professional I became later in my career, and influenced my business style and professionalism after working with her for two short years. I equally impressed her because I became the youngest female board member of the Oswego Alumni Association at that time when I left employment to get married and move. To be respected as the youngest female board member meant I needed to look and dress the part and contribute on a high conversational level to prove my worth, which was easy to do with Olive and Peg as role models.

Not all women have such wonderful relationships with other women, so I count myself blessed. Looking deeply at the women in my life story, there is one thread weaving through all the female relationships. Every woman looks good, dresses well, works passionately in their career, are fun-loving and kind to others.

If I sound as if the most important thing that matters is the outside appearances, achievements and styles of women, then you might assume that's all that matters to me. It is not what inspires me about people but unfortunately what seems to matter in today's American society. Do you believe you are equally concerned about your appearance and the way people perceive you so that you are accepted in work and public? Isn't it true that having a certain look is the American standard in the media and the reason women are always on diets, having surgery or trying to stay fit? I remember once being asked by a therapist why I was so vain, and I replied, "I don't think I'm vain, I just want to look good like the examples set by the women in my life."

CHAPTER O

Overcoming Obstacles

When I left my job in Oswego to marry and move with my husband, I not only needed to change my address and phone number, but hairdressers. Once women have a trusted hairdresser, it is hard to change and trust someone else. Fortunately for me, my mother had an electric, quirky, beautiful hairdresser named Michalle cutting her hair, so I visited her for an appointment. Michalle was on the cutting edge of hair design and colors, traveling often to New York City from Central New York to learn the best techniques to color and style hair. Like most good hairdressers, Michalle listened to my stories each visit and transformed my long straight hair that looked like Karen Carpenter to Whitney Houston's curly tresses. I loved my hair, especially when the wind swirled it around my face.

One day while Michalle was cutting my hair she said, "Tracy, you have a quarter-size bald patch under your thick dark curls." I said, "Oh, that's strange. I've never had anything like that before." She said, "I think it's alopecia." When I arrived home, I called my mom and asked her about it. She told me my father had the same issue as a senior in college, but it healed after he finished exams. "You must be stressed like your father was in college," my mom said. I decided to visit a doctor to confirm the diagnosis. Sure enough, it was a sign of alopecia, an autoimmune disorder where white blood cells attack healthy hair cells thinking they are a foreign body. The immune cells don't recognize healthy hair cells as good cells, they think they are bad and attack them. Since the spot was only a quarter-size, the doctor was not alarmed and sent me home with steroid foam which helped my hair regrow.

By age thirty, I was running my own event planning and management company and juggling motherhood with two young sons, when a few more alopecia spots appeared, making me assume I was stressed again. As a quarter-size spot grew into an area the size of my palm, concern crept in. On the horizon was a high-end wedding on the lawn of a client's lakefront property. This client was a perfectionist and I was concerned my hair condition would be seen and would be bothersome to him. Fortunately, the spot stayed concealed under my locks. Thankfully, the wedding was a grand success and no one noticed my hair. In time it grew back just like my client's green lawn after the wedding guests trampled the grass down,

Another ten years lapsed as I joyfully bounced around with healthy hair until my beloved father died unexpectedly. With his loss, came the loss of 80% of my hair. It fell out like autumn leaves being whipped off trees in a storm. I knew it had to be stress or loss that stripped me of my beautiful brown locks. Devastated, I sought help from an alopecia specialist an hour away from my home and even traveled to Boston to consult with another specialist. Both doctors agreed a heavy dose of oral steroids combined with steroid shots to my head would work, but my hair would take time to grow back fully. The fun fact about hair is it only grows one inch a month, so when you have none, it takes a couple years to get it back to shoulder length, which is what I had before losing the majority of it.

Not convinced my hair loss was totally from alopecia, a few loved ones insisted I have an entire medical review from top to bottom to rule out anything else. After suggesting this to my doctor, she scheduled me for a CT scan to image my brain since some bloodwork levels came back elevated. I will never forget my doctor calling me when the results came in announcing on a voice mail message that the images showed a small micro-adenoma tumor and five-inch cyst in my brain. In the movies, when you hear someone say they see their life flash before their eyes, believe them. It happened to me the minute my doctor told me my condition as my three-year-old son stood between my legs. Everything spun before my eyes including my past, present and perhaps future, my son without his mother. It was devastating news for a week until my doctor sent me to a neurosurgeon for a consultation.

Since I come from a family of doctors, including my uncle and two cousins, I called them immediately for their advice. Because of the influence of growing up in a medical family, I was never scared or intimidated by doctors. They seemed approachable and I always acted as my own best health care advocate. I often wished I had gone into the medical field but didn't have the money or desire to fund an eight year education after my bachelor's degree. Instead, I read and learned everything about my diagnosis so that I was informed when speaking to professional health care providers. I knew my body like no one else did and if I could harness that knowledge and communicate it well to doctors, I was confident in regaining my health.

CHAPTER 5

Solitude

E ventually the neurosurgeon confirmed both growths were non-malignant with the 5" cyst most likely there since birth. The small tumor could be treated with medicine and wouldn't cause an issue. I remember the neurosurgeon saying, "You'll know if your tumor grows because you'll have the worst headache of your life. Similar to falling in love for the first time—you will know!" I left his office hoping I would never feel Cupid's arrow strike me in the head. I wondered if they taught neurosurgeons about love in medical school since that was his best advice. I was relieved surgery wasn't needed because I was afraid the doctor would remove the feminist part of my brain, changing my career mission and life passion forever.

I decided to listen to the wise words and love from my family and announced to my expanding business customers I was taking a three-month medical sabbatical to take care of myself, allowing time for more tests and ensuring the hair loss wasn't related to stress. It was the hardest day of my life to send the email message to one hundred women entre-preneurs telling them I was walking away from my business.

I could never imagine the beautiful replies filling my inbox while taking a long walk. Upon my return, the inbox was full of 90 positive messages. The compassion I felt from my members to take as much time as I needed was overwhelming. With their support, I could take care of myself and return someday to my business healthier than before.

During those three months, I maintained my weekly inspirational newsletter called "The Wednesday Wisdom" to stay connected to them. I did not perform any live events which might stress my body or mind. Instead I strolled through the park, swam in our pool or visited out-of-town family members, resting as best I could to ensure my hair and health returned one day, while taking a heavy round of steroids which had been successful for other alopecia patients.

Sharing a personal story of illness opened my eyes to the compassionate nature of people. I wasn't looking for sympathy in my honesty, I was trying to be an effective business leader to clients who deserved to know why I wouldn't be working for three months. What I received in return was the compassion I needed to confidently walk away and take care of myself. Did I lose business during my sabbatical? If I did, I didn't notice, because I knew business would be there when I returned. Health took priority over career.

CHAPTER E

Empathy and Entrepreneurship

When women start companies, they educate themselves with business courses in sales, marketing, finance and planning. Nowhere in their studies do they find information and advice on dealing with unexpected personal challenges that arise in long-lasting businesses. Personal difficulties such as coping with aging parents, finding daycare solutions, dealing with unexpected medical emergencies, handling the death of loved ones or divorcing a mate are situations that appear in entrepreneurs' lives requiring personal attention and time away from the office.

One time at a business event for women entrepreneurs, a presenter asked the audience to write down the top reason they left a paying job to start their companies. Like most people, I assumed they would say to make unlimited income and earn more salary than at a traditional job. To my surprise, the number one reason women in the room choose entrepreneurship was for flexibility. They desired freedom and flexibility to mesh their personal and career responsibilities.

Flexibility made perfect sense to me since I started my first business when my sons were three years old and three months old so I could be a mother and career woman simultaneously. Not many female business owners at that time admitted to running their companies out of their homes afraid to be discriminated against for not working in a corporate space. Balancing life in my early business years, without abundant technology or revenue, meant taking my sons to the library where I could use new computers, outlining specific times of the day to speak to clients on the phone and booking babysitters when I needed to handle customer appointments out of my home. I never minded the juggling of duties because I was crafting a well-balanced life.

During my bouts with alopecia, the most understanding people besides my family were customers and business associates. The empathy I felt from them made me comfortable walking away from work to rest and recover until it was time to re-enter the workplace more energized because of their support and improved health. Sharing this wisdom with other women business owners became a passion of mine upon returning to work full-time. Taking phone calls or lunch appointments with other female business owners provided me the opportunity to inspire them to also take time away from their companies making their physical or mental health a priority.

CHAPTER H

Healing and Humor

Laughter cures most everything, and so can therapy. In the height of losing my hair and at the suggestion of a close friend, I started seeing a therapist to make sure I wasn't stressed overall which she believed led to the alopecia. Shortly after securing a therapist, my dermatologist told me to brace myself, because

I would be bald in a month if the steroids didn't work. I remember sobbing as I walked out of her office, while checking out of the parking garage and on the entire one-hour ride home as the summer breeze blew through the few strands of hair left on my head, all while a melancholy Carpenters song played on the radio. I didn't want to be bald. I didn't want to lose my business, my husband, my sons or anyone else in my life if I lost all my hair. I drove straight to my therapist's office and exclaimed boldly to her, "I can lose all my hair, but I won't lose my love and passion to help women entrepreneurs! I will fight this! I will keep my business! I will have hair! I will keep going!" Tenacious Tracy took control.

Like women diagnosed with breast cancer using chemotherapy to combat the disease, most admit losing their hair is the hardest part of the journey. For most of them, their hair eventually comes back, typically curly. I decided to purchase a $2,000 real hair wig, perfectly matching the color and cut of my old hair style and covering 80% of my head that was bald while hair was slowly growing back. I needed the wig to wear at professional events being planned and hosted by my company.

One day as I sat at my son's lacrosse game in a ferocious wind, praying my wig wouldn't fly off into the face of another parent, I decided it was time to show up at the next game without a wig with only new short curly hair. Everyone was shocked by my appearance, thinking I cut, permed and dyed my hair within a day, until I explained that a wig had covered my head for six months. Just like a fairy tale, my hair returned in its long beautiful glory in two years.

I enjoyed every ounce of that long hair, washing it gently, letting it blow in the breeze and never allowing myself to say I had a bad hair day. It wasn't possible to have a bad hair day because I had hair! My dermatologist had been wrong about losing it all which made me ecstatic. It wasn't until ten years later after slowing growing all my hair back, that I started losing it again this time after my wonderful stepmother J.B. tragically slipped away due to Alzheimer's disease on the first day of spring. Six months following her death, my hair fell out faster than the first time as the disease spun out of control again.

Knowing a medical sabbatical helped me the first time, I immediately took another one to hide the issue, allowing myself time to grieve and get rebalanced. Mornings were spent doing activities like praying, yoga, meditation, swimming, running, biking, writing and even painting. 100% of the time, Dave Matthews Band music accompanied me, making me happy and positive while listening to their songs. But this time, unlike the first bad bout of alopecia, I was also going through menopause, which made the condition worse. Women talk about hot flashes, night sweats, gaining weight, and moodiness during menopause, but no one talks about thinning hair. I think this stage of life, in addition to my genetic disposition to alopecia and the loss of my dear stepmother of 42 years, made it rain hair.

I remember finding comfort in my husband's arms, crying because my instincts indicated this time was different. Although I tried new treatments, like having my blood drawn monthly, mixed with a serum and then injected back into my head (50 shots at a cost of $500 each time), and new topical products, along with another round of oral steroids, and shampoo that promised hair growth, but nothing worked. Before all the leaves fell off the trees, I only had a tiny ponytail of hair. Everyone told me to cut it off but I had a feeling if I did, it might never come back.

One morning, feeling brave, I went into the bathroom, grabbed my husband's scissors and cut the ponytail off! I had little tuffs of hair sporadically on my head like tumbleweed bunches spotted in the desert landscape. Cutting off of the pony tail made me feel free and rebellious. I remember fingering my short hair and being excited I did it. I was content with short hair for the first time in my life until my premonition came true and a change in a long-term medicine made the little hair I had left fall out. I was a bald woman for the first time in my life at the age of 54.

Thankfully born with a great sense of humor because of my parents who at any time could set me on a laughing attack because of their jokes, antics and slapstick form of comedy, I used humor to cope with my new found baldness.

A fun fact about steroids, which I took every time I lost a majority of my hair, is while it's growing your hair, it is also reshaping a regular-looking face into a full-moon-shaped face with hair on it; all while adding ten pounds to your frame. In the midst of my steroid transformation, I stood at the kitchen counter one morning next to my husband when I looked at him and then looked back at myself and said, "Wow, we are starting to look alike! I'm growing hair on my face like you! I'm gaining weight and approaching your weight. And now you have man boobs as big as my chest!" Our sons will come downstairs and say, "Hey, which one is Mom and which one is Dad?" My husband and I laughed until tears rolled down our cheeks because what else could we do.

In another instance, a dear friend stopped by for a poolside chat and swim. No one had seen my bald head besides my family so I was perplexed on how to manage her visit since swimming was involved. I decided to greet her with a rose-colored baseball hat on and take it off once I was ready to submerge in the aqua water. As she tipped-toed in the cool pool water, I jumped in completely. Slowly emerging upwards and stopping only enough to showoff the top of my head, I stayed there for a minute. As I reappeared on the surface within earshot of my friend, I said, "Guess what I just was?" She didn't know. I said, "A buoy! Do you get it?" I used that same joke many times afterwards getting giggles and belly laughs from visitors and family members.

As Halloween approached later that year, knowing it was a perfect opportunity to disguise myself in a unique costume, I contemplated dressing up as "Mr. Clean," the "Magic 8 Ball" or "Charlie Brown." I finally settled on replicating Uncle Fester from "The Addams Family."

All I needed was a tan trench coat, dark circles around my eyes and a bald head. Although my comedic tendencies seemed self-deprecating, my family was thrilled to see me finding a silver lining with my condition and so was I.

CHAPTER A

Acceptance

If you could stop reading for a moment and look at the pre- and post-alopecia photos of me in this book on page 104, you'll notice my face is pretty much the same. The only thing missing is my hair, eyebrows and eyelashes. If it was winter, you'd see my nose running, because alopecia strips away nose hair and nose hair indicates to someone their nose is about to run. I never knew a nose could run so fast and undetectable, like water from a pipe, before I experienced it for the first time. If you were up close and touched my forearm you would think I have the softest skin in America, too. You know why? When you don't have hair on your arms, your skin feels smooth, and so do your legs. This is the only bonus that comes with alopecia!

I hope you ask yourself right now what is similar or different about me since you began reading this book? Here is some wisdom I have gleaned.

- Internally I am still the same woman minus thick dark hair, long eyelashes, and eyebrows, so I appear different in the mirror and to others.

- My life experiences are the same as they were before I lost all my hair.

- I am still vain, which means I care what other people think of my looks. I realized over time that I wear my wigs for other people and not for myself and I wear them to conform to society when it is necessary.

- I tell every woman I meet to never complain about having a bad hair day because that's not possible until you experience complete baldness. Love your hair and be gentler with yourself when gazing in the mirror. Be less critical of others who might not look as put-together as society expects.

- I also realize participating in sports allows me to be free to be bald because no one running or biking cares if a bald woman is running or biking next to them because they are totally focused on their own sporting experience.

Since I have always worn my company's brand colors, especially the color rose and pink for women, and since I serve female entrepreneurs, I started wearing different shades of rose-colored hats after becoming bald when participating in sports, working outside or running errands. Wearing a hat was the only option since it is impossible to wear a wig during hot summer temperatures and humidity.

The rose-colored hat also identified me as a woman, since many men called me "Sir," to my dismay, when I wore a blue or black hat. I also pierced my ears to appear more feminine and wore more necklaces and bracelets. Anything I could do to look more attractive, I did. I just wanted strangers to see me as a female.

The tagline for my company, Women TIES, became "Women Supporting Women in Business, Sports, Equality, and Life" in 2017 when I trained for the Boston Marathon. When you run ten or more miles, your mind wanders, and this tagline spoke to me one day. I eventually put the tagline on my marketing materials, shirts and rose-colored hats.

But when I wore any shade of pink hat, which displayed the absence of hair, eyebrows and eyelashes, people assumed I had cancer. Sympathic looks from strangers, people unexpectedly getting up and giving me their seat, letting me go ahead of them in line, holding the door open, unexpectedly hugging me, and praying for me, were common. I even got to cut in front of a woman in line for confessions at church on Good Friday. I often wonder if it was because I looked sick or if she needed one more good deed before heading in to confess.

I also felt guilty when people were overly nice to me, not asking what illness I had, but assuming it was serious. I was not lying about the severity of my medical condition by not hiding under a wig, tattooing my eyebrows or wearing false eyelashes, but most times these generous people were the ones who needed or wanted to give the support. The quote "in giving we receive" is very evident in my everyday interactions with people who look at me as a bald woman.

CHAPTER T

Togetherness

The best insight I experienced, saw, felt, and heard from wearing my rose-colored hats is actually the meaning of the color pink itself, which is unconditional love. Unconditional love of oneself by accepting the way we look today because we age every day of our lives. Showing unconditional love to others struggling with their own appearance, illness or non-society-accepting trait and love from others who go out of their way to be kind because they assume, I am ill by my appearance.

I think in today's world with so much bitterness, divide and anger over political differences, religious beliefs, sexual orientation, ethnicity, and origin of birth, people have forgotten that unconditional love and kindness is necessary and so simple to give. It doesn't cost anything and only requires an open heart, mind and generous spirit.

Every year attending the New York State Fair I sit somewhere long enough to watch everyday people walk by, while identifying something beautiful about them, even if society might not agree. It could be someone's light green eyes, a simple necklace, their stature or shoes, a hairstyle or even their sun-kissed skin. I always find something I like about every person I see. I do this because I want to find something beautiful about everyone. I choose to look at others knowing they are beautiful in some way. Sometimes it might not be the beautiful image found on magazine covers, in films or after the beauty shop, but it is the unique essence of every person. We each have something about us or inside us that is beautiful and it takes unconditional, universal love to recognize and act on it.

Parking my car one blustery April day, to head into a bank to get money to go to Boston to run in my first marathon, the wind was blowing hard. As a frail woman came out of the bank doors, a big gust of wind almost blew her over. Witnessing the alarm in her eyes, I approached to see if she needed help getting to her car. She nodded yes, so I extended my arm for her to grasp, but instead she interlaced her fingers into mine, like a boyfriend and girlfriend in the beginning of a relationship. We walked gingerly towards her car hand in hand. By the time we got to her door, I shared the fact I was withdrawing money to travel to Massachusetts to run the Boston Marathon. She said, "What's your name?" I told her "Tracy." She said, "Well, Tracy, I am going to pray you are successful in the race because of your kindness today." I gave her a hug, closed her door once her feet were tucked inside, and went into the bank smiling. I love being kind to strangers.

This feeling of kindness must have traveled with me to Boston, because two nights before the race, worried about completing it, I stopped eating. I knew I needed food to fuel my 26.2-mile run, so I walked to a pizza parlor and bought a medium pizza pie and salad. I sat down and ate only a quarter of the pizza and salad, figuring I would save the rest for later. As I walked back to my hotel, I came upon a man looking through a trashcan for food to eat. I walked over to him without a thought and asked him if he wanted my warm pizza. He accepted my gift, thanking me. Not unlike the beggar in the Jim Carrey movie "Bruce Almighty," where the city beggar morphed from his ragged look into God played by Morgan Freeman, this Boston man could have been God or just a hungry man needing food. All I wanted to be was kind in the moment.

In another instance, leaving a café with my good friend Shannon, I wore a rose-colored hat to cover my bald head when a woman got up from her seat and rushed across the café straight to me saying, "I was just diagnosed with cancer." Her eyes welled with tears and her expression grim. I said, "What kind of cancer do you have?" She said, "Bile Duct Cancer in two places. What do you have?" I said gently, "I don't have cancer, I have alopecia. But I love hugging women who need hugs and you look like you need one!" as I gently pulled her into my arms and wished her well. Once outside, my friend said, "Tracy, that must be hard for you, always having people think you have cancer." I responded, "It isn't if I can help, comfort or support them in some way by acknowledging their sadness, worry or despair and give them whatever they need in the moment; I'm happy to do so." I honestly think God paused my life because he wants me to share this lesson of unconditional love and kindness with others.

I realize now my rose-colored hat is like a beacon of light shining for others to find unconditional love and support by sharing their own or a loved one's health story with me or to simply show kindness and love to a stranger because it makes them feel better. Not unlike my female relatives, giving love and compassion is the secret joy of life.

Four valuable messages, from wearing the rose-colored hat, are important to share with you.

First, the rose-colored hat attracts people or their loved ones to me who have an illness like cancer or alopecia so *they can share their story* at the moment they feel like expressing it to a stranger. God has a plan for me and everyone when tough times happen. For me it is to share the empathy and kindness I've witnessed over my life and especially during my alopecia story. I know if you are faced with difficulty, you will also find the meaning of your trials. Pause and let the answer come to you.

Second, the rose-colored hat allows me to embrace women with breast cancer or people with a cancer diagnosis. Most people associate the color pink with breast cancer awareness, and through my company, Women TIES, I meet four to five women each year who are diagnosed, recovering, battling a second diagnosis of the disease or who are in remission. Two decades of running a business, dedicated to helping women, means women in my circles reveal they had or have it. The statistics startle me. Wearing a rose-colored hat also opens up the breast cancer and cancer conversations. The hat gets me noticed and triggers the right conversations with the right people who need it.

Third, since my entrepreneurial career is focused on supporting women, the rose-colored hat gives me the opportunity to share my message of "Women Supporting Women in Business, Sports, Equality, and Life." The rose-colored hat makes me stand out in a crowd where I have a chance to share my mission of women buying from women first and foremost to help strengthen the financial buying circle for females until an equality pay law is passed in America.

Finally, the rose-colored hat makes me feel comfortable with myself when that's what I need most after becoming bald. To feel good in one's own skin is essential for a happy life; it doesn't matter if one doesn't meet society's norms.

Conclusion

Hopefully, looking again at my headshots, you can identify me as the same woman, because I am the identical woman since the first page of this book with the same message, voice, height, weight, heart and brain. No matter if I wear makeup or not, have hair or not, dress up or dress down, wear heels or run in sneakers, my appearance shouldn't matter. What's most important about every single woman, man, girl or boy in this world, is who they are on the inside.

Society and beauty norms might make you believe differently, but you have heard me debunk that myth by describing myself in the beginning of the book with a full head of real hair to a bald woman wearing a sporty rose-colored hat. Nothing else changed in my appearance or person, just what was on top of my head and possibly other's perception of me once my looks changed.

The person I see in the mirror now might not look like the same woman a couple years ago, but she is there; she can't leave and won't be forgotten, because the most important part of who we are is the good, kind person we choose to be on the inside. Your heart, spirit and compassionate, loving thoughts towards yourself and others is what matters most of all.

I hope if you see anyone with any type of disability, difference in skin color or hair color, height, weight, type of clothes, car or career, or social standing that you treat them with kindness and love.

I still wish with all my heart I had hair, but I have also learned how kind people are when I look different from them. I try to be a sympathetic, inspirational, upbeat woman willing to help others because it doesn't take a head of hair to be that; it takes a giving heart, which in my opinion makes you more beautiful, different and special than anything you can put on or fix about your appearance.

So, if you are faced with self-doubt, comparing yourself to others for any reason at all, remember the messages under the rose-colored hat. Life is about being kind and accepting yourself, with the normal and not-so-normal parts of yourself that make you exactly who you are meant to be—YOU! Wear it proud. If you are a girl, wear your pink, especially your rose-colors! Be kind to others, and most importantly, be kind and love yourself! If we can't be our own best friend, treating ourselves with love and compassion because we deserve it, no one else will.

Inspiration

Since I found healing and joy by the sea in beloved Sanibel Island, after dealing with my alopecia diagnosis for two years, I leave this inspirational thought to inspire healing in your life too.

Life goes on through personal difficulties. Although we feel barren inside and out with worry, light still surrounds us. We are never alone when we have love and great joy of what was. When our spirit becomes low and everyday circumstances seem difficult, reclaim your peace of mind through joyful recollections of the past believing happiness is right around the corner.

Just like finding new seashells on every beach walk, there are new daily insights in every tough situation. The ocean tide surges twice a day and so can the joys and difficulties in life when dealing with suffering of some kind, but one afternoon the sun's glow shines on your cheeks, soft sand soothes your toes, and a colorful dune flower brightens your view bringing you back to wholeness.

Each step on a healing journey is one of realization and acceptance. No one knows when they are ready to emerge from the dark until that one glorious ray awakens the spirit to start living fully again. We wait patiently for the right time to emerge whole, trusting it will come and joy will follow.

Blessings,
Tracy

Acknowledgements

This book easily poured out of my heart because of the amazing people who have graced my life and the compassionate strangers, through brief life-changing encounters, who inspired me to share the kindness that exists in the world.

This book wouldn't be possible without my husband Scott Higginbotham who loves my writing. When we renewed our marital vows on our 30th wedding anniversary in Sanibel Island, Florida, a wig adorned my bald head. He has loved me unconditionally, with and without hair, and his love renewed my belief and love in myself after two difficult years of physical transformation.

My sons Thomas Higginbotham and Adam Higginbotham have always accepted my feminist spirit, athletic loves and my newfound baldness. Their love enriches my life every day. They are true blessings from above.

To my Mother Patricia Rickard-Lauri, thank you for passing down my spunky, independent, feminist, athletic genes and providing an upbringing that empowered me to achieve all the things I have done as a woman entrepreneur. I am grateful for my deep love for fitness, cooking, writing and nature which came from you.

I couldn't write this book without heavenly guidance from my wonderful Father Chuck Chamberlain and Stepmother J.B. Chamberlain who reside in my heart forever. Dad, thank you for giving me an amazing sense of humor that helped me deal with alopecia with grace and laughs. I know you were laughing with me at my side and hugging me when I was crying. Heaven isn't far away.

Thank you to my awe-inspiring aunts Elaine Amidon and Dona Maroney and grandmothers Minnie Lauri and Ginny Chamberlain who showed me abundant love in their lifetimes and molded me into a kind and compassionate woman from their affectionate examples.

Leadership started when I was designated the oldest sibling of a mixed, loving bunch of eight kids. To my sister Jill Chamberlain Delviscio, thank you for a lifetime of unconditional love and support. I couldn't have asked for a better girl to go through life with especially with all its twists and turns. To Christine Gerber, Marlana Scott and Elizabeth Phillips, you are my real sisters forever. To Bre Chamberlain, Chad Chamberlain and Jake Chamberlain, I love you like you are my own children. I'm here for all of you always.

Fifty years of my life has been filled with the friendship, humor and deep love of my friend Lynda Rolston Krause. I can't thank her enough for believing in me and funding this book. We are soul sisters forever. Equally, I thank Geselle DeMatteo Sadler, who has been my other best friend. Someday we'll have those walks together as we talk about.

Thank you to my spiritual friend Teresa Dowe Huggins for providing me with peaceful retreats, lunch discussions and pink visions of this book. You are an amazing friend and believer in all things that are good and positive.

I became fearless when I met Kathrine Switzer. Her exuberant personality and zest for life taught me to take risks I wouldn't have taken including running in the 2017 Boston Marathon with her and Team 261Fearless.

Thank you to my husband's family for always supporting my endeavors and showing concern and love while dealing with my illness. I am blessed with wonderful in-laws.

A special acknowledgement to two women who helped this book become a reality with their expertise in publishing and editing – Sharon CassanoLochman and Tracy Black. I couldn't have done this without you.

To my loyal and dedicated Women TIES Advisory Board of Directors Shannon Magari, Karen McMahon, Joan Powers, and Gwen Webber-McLeod thanks for 15 years of advice, support and belief in me and my company.

The Dave Matthews Band plays in my ears everyday so I have to thank them for their infectious music I run, bike, work, drive and write to every day since 1999. The songs simply fill me with joy. Thank you for the song "Everyday" that inspired me on the toughest days during my medical condition.

Finally, for any past or present Women TIES members, thank you for believing in my vision in women doing business with women first and foremost and putting your money in the hands, pocketbooks and bank accounts of women owned businesses until women finally earn the same as men. With your support in my personal and corporate career mission, we are financially changing the world for women.

Services Available

Tracy Chamberlain Higginbotham speaks to audiences all over the country particularly in topics related to women entrepreneurs, work-at-home mothers and women needing to take a break from their careers for their health. Tracy is expanding her speaking topics to include lessons learned under the rose-colored hat. Potential audiences include, but are not limited to, people dealing with alopecia or life changing health issues or people whose appearance doesn't fit society's normal standards.

Tracy will also be spreading the message of kindness, compassion and acceptance of others across the country to help heal divides and fractions sowed at this time in our nation's history.

Because many young people dealing with alopecia are bullied, just like many children and teenagers in today's culture when they are ridiculed for looking or behaving differently, Tracy wants to address this demographic to enlighten and lift them up with her message.

For further information on Tracy Chamberlain Higginbotham or to secure her for a speaking opportunity, visit: www.tracyhigginbotham.com or www.womenties.com or call 315-708-4288.

About the Author

Tracy Chamberlain Higginbotham is the Founder and President of Women TIES, LLC (aka: Women Together Inspiring Entrepreneurial Success) a company created in 2005 that specializes in promoting, publicizing and uniting women entrepreneurs and their companies online and in person in order to cultivate strong economic relationships to advance their companies and eradicate pay inequality.

She became a woman entrepreneur in 1995 by creating her first company Five Star Events, an events management company she ran for 15 years. In 2005, Tracy embraced her passion for supporting other women entrepreneurs and established her second company, Women TIES, LLC.

In 2011, Tracy created a division of Women TIES called the "Women's Athletic Network" which promotes athletic events for women entrepreneurs to participate in, train for or support as spectators. In 2017, Higginbotham also created a "Women's Equality" division to Women TIES to unite women who are interested in being more involved with equality issues for women. Tracy believes strongly in "Women supporting women in business, sports, equality and life."

Higginbotham is a 1986 graduate of the State University of New York at Oswego where she earned a Bachelor of Science degree in Business Administration and post graduate studies in Business Management.

Tracy's dedication to supporting women entrepreneurship was recognized by the Small Business Administration twice – once in 2005 and again in 2011 when she received the Region II "Women Owned Business Champion Award." The Women Business Champion award is given to someone for their significant contributions as an outstanding small business person and for dedicated support of small business.

She was the columnist of the Syracuse Post Standard's "Ask the Entrepreneur" column for 11 years. She has written an inspirational e-newsletter for women entrepreneurs for 15 years. Higginbotham is also a published writer whose inspirational short stories and articles appear in several national publications and books, including the 2009 "Chicken Soup for the Soul: Power Moms" and the 2019 "Chicken Soup for the Soul: Running for Good."

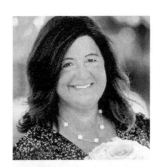

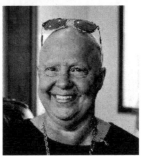

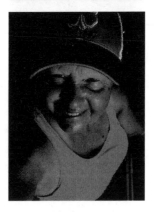

Made in the USA
Lexington, KY
30 November 2019